Extraction technicians

Understanding the roles Extraction technicians play in the filed of chemical engineering

Dr Walt wade

Contents

chapter1

introduction to extraction technician

Extraction technicians play a crucial role in the field of chemical engineering and are an integral part of the extraction industry. They are responsible for extracting, purifying, and isolating various substances from raw materials through various extraction processes. Extraction, also known as the separation process, is the process of removing a desired compound or substance from a mixture. It is a critical step in the production of chemicals, pharmaceuticals, and other industrial products. Extraction technicians work in a laboratory setting, carefully following established protocols and procedures to ensure the extraction process is efficient and safe. An extraction technician must have a deep understanding of chemistry, chemical engineering principles, and laboratory techniques. They must also possess strong analytical skills and be able to work with precision and attention to detail. Being an extraction technician requires a high level of expertise and an aptitude for solving complex problems. There are various types of extraction techniques, each with its own unique process and purpose. Some of the most commonly used techniques include solid-liquid extraction, liquid-liquid extraction, and supercritical fluid extraction. Solid-liquid extraction involves the separation of a solid compound from a liquid. This technique is commonly used in the production of pharmaceuticals and nutraceuticals. Liquid-liquid extraction, also known as solvent extraction, is the process of isolating a desired substance from a liquid mixture by using a solvent. This technique is used in the production of essential oils, flavors, and fragrances. Supercritical fluid extraction is a newer technique that uses a supercritical fluid, such as carbon dioxide, to extract compounds from solid or liquid materials. This technique is environmentally friendly and is often used in the extraction of natural substances from plants and herbs. Extraction technicians must also have a thorough understanding of the properties and behaviors of different chemicals and substances. They must be able to identify the most appropriate extraction method for a specific compound or mixture, and adjust and optimize the extraction conditions to obtain the best results. In addition to being responsible for the extraction process, technicians also play a crucial role in the purification and isolation of extracted compounds. This involves using various techniques such as distillation, filtration, and chromatography to separate, purify, and concentrate the desired substance. One of the critical skills of an extraction technician is the ability to use and maintain various laboratory equipment and instruments. They must be proficient in using tools such as centrifuges, rotary evaporators, and analytical instruments like gas chromatographs and mass spectrometers. These instruments are essential for monitoring and analyzing the extraction process and ensuring the purity and quality of the final product. Safety is of utmost importance in the extraction industry, and technicians must understand and adhere to all safety protocols and procedures. They must be trained and knowledgeable about handling hazardous chemicals, wearing protective gear, and following correct disposal methods. A small error in handling chemicals can lead to significant safety hazards, which is why a thorough understanding of safety measures is crucial for an extraction technician. Apart from technical skills, extraction technicians also need to have excellent communication and teamwork skills. They often work in collaboration with other scientists and engineers, and clear communication is essential to ensure the success of the extraction process. As the field of extraction continues to evolve and new and innovative techniques are developed, technicians must also be willing to adapt and learn new methods and technologies. In conclusion, extraction technicians play a vital role in the extraction industry by using their in-depth knowledge of chemistry, laboratory techniques, and equipment to extract, purify, and isolate various compounds from raw materials. Their role in the production of chemicals, pharmaceuticals, and other industrial products is crucial, and their expertise is fundamental to ensure the safety and quality of the final product. With the demand for these skills increasing, the role of an extraction technician is becoming more important than ever in the field of chemical engineering.

chapter2

extraction technician salary

Extraction technicians are an essential part of the cannabis industry, playing a key role in the production of high-quality cannabis products. As the demand for cannabis products continues to increase, the demand for skilled extraction technicians has also risen. This has led to a surge in job opportunities in this field, with attractive salaries being offered to those who possess the necessary expertise and experience. The primary responsibility of an extraction technician is to extract cannabinoids and other desirable compounds from the cannabis plant, using various extraction methods such as butane, CO_2, or ethanol. Their role is crucial in ensuring that the extracted concentrate is of high quality, safe for consumption, and free from any impurities or contaminants. One of the main factors that determine the salary of an extraction technician is their level of experience. In general, entry-level extraction technicians with limited experience can expect to earn an average annual salary of $30,000 to $40,000 in the United States. This may increase to $50,000 to $60,000 per year for those with a few years of experience. Apart from experience, the location of the job also plays a significant role in determining the salary of an extraction technician. In states where cannabis is legal, there is a higher demand for extraction technicians, and as a result, the salaries tend to be higher. According to a survey by Cannabis Business Times, the average salary of an extraction technician in states where cannabis is legal is around $47,000, while in states where it is still illegal, the average salary is around $39,000. Another factor that contributes to the salary of an extraction technician is their level of education and training. Although there is no formal education requirement for this position, having a degree in chemistry or a related field can lead to higher pay. Additionally, more extensive training and certifications in extraction techniques can also increase an extraction technician's salary. The type of company or organization an extraction technician works for can also impact their salary. Extraction technicians who work for large, established cannabis companies or research institutions tend to earn higher salaries compared to those working for small startups or businesses. This is because larger companies have more resources to invest in their employees and can offer better pay and benefits. In addition to their base salary, many extraction technicians also receive bonuses or incentives based on their performance. For example, if they are able to consistently produce high-quality extracts with high yields, they may receive monetary bonuses or promotions. This is a common practice in the cannabis industry and can significantly increase an extraction technician's annual income. With the growing popularity of cannabis products, the demand for extraction technicians is expected to continue to rise, and along with it, their salaries. As the industry becomes more established and regulations become clearer, there will be an increased need for skilled and experienced extraction technicians, which will further drive up their salaries. Apart from the salary, extraction technicians also receive other benefits such as health insurance, paid time off, and retirement plans. In states where cannabis is legal, many companies also offer stock options or equity in the company, which can add significant value to an extraction technician's compensation package. Moreover, as the cannabis industry continues to evolve, extraction technicians are not limited to just working for cannabis companies. They can also use their skills and knowledge to work in other related industries such as food and beverage, pharmaceuticals, and cosmetics. These industries also offer competitive salaries and benefits, providing more opportunities for extraction technicians.

chapter3

extraction technician job description

Job Responsibilities: 1. Conducting preliminary surveys and site evaluations: Extraction technicians are responsible for conducting thorough surveys and evaluations of potential oil and gas extraction sites. This involves analyzing geographical and geological data, assessing the feasibility of extraction, and conducting risk assessments. 2. Designing and implementing extraction processes: Based on their evaluations, technicians design and implement extraction processes that are specific to each site. This includes selecting appropriate extraction methods, designing equipment and infrastructure, and ensuring compliance with safety regulations. 3. Operating and maintaining extraction equipment: Extraction technicians are responsible for the proper operation and maintenance of equipment used in the extraction process. This includes pumps, compressors, separators, and other machinery used to extract and process the hydrocarbons. 4. Monitoring and controlling extraction processes: Technicians must constantly monitor and control the extraction process to ensure that it runs smoothly and efficiently. They use various tools and instruments to monitor pressure, temperature, and other parameters, and make adjustments as needed. 5. Troubleshooting: In case of any issues during the extraction process, technicians must quickly identify and troubleshoot the problem to minimize downtime. This requires a strong understanding of the equipment and processes being used. 6. Ensuring safety and compliance: Extraction technicians must strictly adhere to safety procedures and regulations to prevent accidents and protect the environment. They are also responsible for ensuring that all processes and operations comply with government regulations and industry standards. 7. Record-keeping and reporting: Technicians are required to maintain detailed records of all extraction activities, including production rates, equipment performance, and any incidents or accidents that occur. They must also prepare reports for management and regulatory agencies as needed. 8. Participating in training and development programs: As technology and extraction methods continue to evolve, extraction technicians must keep up with new developments through training and development programs. They need to constantly upgrade their skills and knowledge to stay abreast of industry advancements. Qualifications and Skills: - A degree in engineering or a related field such as chemical or mechanical engineering is typically required for an extraction technician position. - Strong analytical and problem-solving skills are essential as technicians are required to troubleshoot and make decisions quickly. - Excellent attention to detail and the ability to follow safety procedures and regulations are crucial to ensure the safety of workers and the environment. - Physical stamina is necessary, as technicians may be required to work in remote locations and in challenging weather conditions. - Strong communication skills are needed to effectively convey information to team members and other stakeholders. - Proficiency in the use of tools and equipment, as well as computer skills, are important for monitoring and controlling extraction processes. - Prior experience working in the oil and gas industry is preferred. Work Environment: Extraction technicians primarily work in oil and gas fields, which are often located in remote and isolated areas. They may also work in refineries and processing plants. The working conditions can be physically demanding, involving long hours and exposure to various weather conditions. Technicians may also be required to work in confined spaces, at heights, and in noisy environments. They must always wear appropriate safety gear, including hard hats, goggles, and protective clothing. Career Outlook: The demand for extraction technicians is expected to remain strong in the coming years as global energy demands increase. This job offers potential for career growth, with opportunities to move into supervisory or management roles with experience and further education. As technology advances and new extraction methods are developed, the need for skilled technicians will continue to rise

chaptert4

extraction technician training

Training and education are vital aspects of becoming an extraction technician. Most employers in this field require a minimum of a bachelor's degree in chemistry, biochemistry, pharmaceutical science, or a related field. These degrees provide the theoretical knowledge and practical skills needed to understand the chemistry behind the extraction process. However, a degree is not enough to become an extraction technician; specialized training is also required. Many colleges and universities offer training programs specifically designed for this role. These programs focus on techniques and procedures used in the extraction process, such as solvent selection, chromatography, and distillation. Hands-on training is an essential part of these programs, giving students the opportunity to apply their theoretical knowledge and practice essential skills. Apart from formal education and training, becoming an extraction technician also requires constant learning and updating of skills. This field is constantly evolving, with new technologies and techniques emerging regularly. As such, it is essential for extraction technicians to keep up-to-date with the latest developments in their field through continuing education and training programs. This ensures that they are equipped with the most recent and relevant skills and knowledge to carry out their job effectively. One of the most critical skills that extraction technicians must possess is attention to detail. The extraction process involves working with delicate and sensitive materials, and even the slightest mistake can lead to contamination or the production of an ineffective or harmful product. Hence, extraction technicians must be meticulous and have a keen eye for detail to ensure the safety and quality of the final product. Moreover, extraction technicians should be able to work well under pressure. The extraction process is time-sensitive, and any delay or error can result in significant losses for the company. Therefore, extraction technicians must be able to handle high levels of stress and work efficiently to complete their tasks within strict deadlines. Along with technical skills, extraction technicians also need to possess excellent communication and teamwork skills. The extraction process often involves working in teams, and therefore, effective communication and collaboration are essential to the success of the project. Extraction technicians must be able to communicate clearly and concisely with their team members, as well as other professionals involved in the process, such as scientists and researchers. Another crucial aspect of the training for extraction technicians is safety protocols. As they work with hazardous chemicals and potentially infectious materials, it is vital for extraction technicians to adhere to strict safety procedures. Their training includes learning about the proper use of personal protective equipment, handling and disposing of hazardous materials, and following safety regulations to prevent accidents and ensure a safe working environment. Extraction technicians must also possess problem-solving skills and must be able to think critically and analytically. The extraction process can be complex, and technicians must be able to troubleshoot any issues that may arise during the process. This requires them to have a strong scientific background and the ability to think outside the box to find solutions to problems. Apart from technical and scientific skills, successful extraction technicians also possess certain personal qualities that contribute to their success in this field. These qualities include being detail-oriented, patient, and adaptable. The extraction process can be time-consuming and requires precision and patience, especially during long hours of repetitive tasks. Extraction technicians must also be adaptable and able to handle unexpected changes in the process, such as variations in the raw materials or equipment. In addition to the necessary skills and qualities, proper work ethics are also crucial for an extraction technician. Since they handle sensitive materials and play a crucial role in the production of life-saving drugs, technicians must adhere to strict ethical standards. This includes maintaining confidentiality and following proper ethical guidelines during research and development processes. The demand for skilled extraction technicians is on the rise due to the increasing demand for pharmaceuticals and natural healthcare products. With the ongoing research and development in these fields, the need for well-trained and highly skilled extraction technicians is expected to grow in the future

.solventless extraction course

Solventless extraction is an innovative and rapidly growing technique used in the extraction of concentrated oils and waxes from plants. This method involves a mechanical separation process that does not use any chemical solvents, making it a safer and more environmentally friendly alternative to traditional extraction methods. The process of solventless extraction begins with high-quality plant material, such as cannabis or hemp, that is free of any contaminants or pesticides. This material is then ground or crushed to increase its surface area for efficient extraction. The ground material is then placed in a specialized machine, such as a hydraulic press or rosin press, where heat and pressure are applied to extract the oils and waxes from the plant material. One of the key advantages of solventless extraction is its ability to produce high-quality concentrated oils and waxes without using any chemical solvents, which can leave harmful residues in the final product. This makes it a preferred method for producing clean, pure and potent extracts for medicinal and recreational use. Additionally, solventless extraction also preserves the flavor and aroma of the original plant material, providing a more natural and authentic experience. Solventless extraction is also significantly faster than other methods, with extraction times ranging from a few minutes to a few hours, depending on the type of machine used. This makes it a more efficient option for large-scale production, allowing producers to quickly meet the demands of the market. As the cannabis and hemp industries continue to grow, so does the demand for clean and potent concentrates. Solventless extraction addresses this need by providing a safer and more effective way to produce high-quality extractions. This has led to a rise in popularity and interest in solventless extraction courses, with many individuals and businesses seeking to learn more about this method. One of the main benefits of enrolling in a solventless extraction course is gaining a comprehensive understanding of the entire process, from selecting the right plant material to using different machines and techniques for extraction. These courses are designed to equip individuals with the knowledge and skills necessary to produce high-quality concentrates consistently. Some of the key topics covered in a typical solventless extraction course include the various types of plant material and their properties, the different types of extraction machines available, the optimal temperatures and pressures for extraction, and post-extraction processes such as curing and storage. Students also learn about the importance of proper safety measures when handling plant material and operating extraction machines. This includes wearing protective gear, maintaining clean and sanitary workspace, and ensuring the proper disposal of plant material after extraction. By emphasizing safe and responsible practices, these courses help prevent accidents and promote a healthier work environment. Additionally, enrolling in a solventless extraction course can also provide valuable networking opportunities. These courses often bring together professionals and industry experts, providing students with a platform to exchange ideas, collaborate and learn from one another. This can lead to potential job opportunities and collaborations, especially for those looking to enter the cannabis and hemp industries. Furthermore, as the demand for solventless extracts continues to rise, there is a growing need for skilled and knowledgeable professionals in this field. By completing a solventless extraction course, individuals can position themselves for job opportunities with extraction companies, cannabis and hemp producers, or start their own solventless extraction business. One of the biggest challenges in the extraction industry is staying up-to-date with the latest techniques and technologies. Solventless extraction courses provide a platform for professionals to stay informed about advancements in the field. As this industry evolves, it is crucial for individuals to continuously upgrade their skills and knowledge to remain competitive and meet the evolving demands of the market.

The end